"Fat is not the enemy in your diet. Fat is your friend." – Jimmy Moore

Introduction

In the USA, it seems there is a new "revolutionary diet" concept just about every few months. Sometimes these "diet plans" catch hold and receive massive buzz across the country. Other times they just fizzle out, only to be replaced with the next one, on a never-ending cycle of experimentation.

I believe I have discovered a way off of that carrousel! My revelation comes from having experienced a true lifestyle change, which has affected my entire Being! *I am over two years in now and have never felt more healthy and "Fit"…*

It all started when my wife, who is a dedicated Cross-fit practitioner, as well as an aspiring endurance athlete, asked me to help her follow a Keto Diet plan that her fitness coach was recommending.

Having been through several of her experimentations with different nutritional philosophies, we each knew that it would be easier for her to accomplish her goals if we could both have the same dietary lifestyle. This meant me getting on board.

Even knowing this, and despite being lovingly devoted to my wife, I was quite resistant to "going on a diet". I just haven't ever been interested in following any "diet plan", as I really enjoy eating.

I enjoy eating whatever and whenever I like, without any rules or worries! I have largely been able to get away with this, without terribly noticeable results from my negligent indulgences, for most of my life, or so I thought...

I seem to have been blessed with good genetics, and great metabolism, so my food choices have, in the past, never really affected me too negatively. I have mostly maintained a pretty steady weight, regardless of the different cycles of lifestyle that I have gone through.

Sure, there have been times where I have been heavier than normal (for me), just as there have been times where I've been lighter. The overall average, though, seemed largely consistent for most of my fully grown adult life.

It wasn't until these last couple of years (now approaching mid-40's at the time of this writing) that I began to notice a change in how I feel, and in how my body processes things, after eating certain foods.

My first conscious discovery of, or at least recognition of, how food was affecting me involved an increase in how many times I felt just flat out miserable shortly after consuming meals. Have you ever had a super strong craving for something specific, like say Mexican food?

If you're like me you have, and not only have you felt that craving, but you gave in to satisfying it as well! I can't count the number of times I felt like I just had to have some Mexican Food! I would inevitably indulge, and indulge, and over indulge, and then some!

It never failed, afterwards, that I then felt absolutely miserable for several hours as my body fought to digest all those binged calories, carbs, and sugars. I can recall always thinking, "man that was stupid, why do we pay (going out to nice restaurants and over eating) so much to feel this terrible?!"

I can't recall how many times I've vowed off certain foods in those agonizing hours of bloated bemoaning. I would get so mad at myself for eating that way and causing all the gaseous bloating, but then I'd be right back at it the next time a craving popped up.

That was my cycle for many food types/groups, for many years. Don't even get me started on how I'd act around a tray of freshly baked cookies! (still my #1 weakness to this day! ☺) I would gorge myself to misery! It was a truly silly cycle, but I suspect I'm not the only one who has been there.

So, when my wife introduced me to the concept of Ketosis (key-tow-sis, for we Southerners), I was willing to try it out, if only to help her. I figured I had nothing to lose (but some fat around my waist!), and could even pick up some "brownie points" (we'll have to explore the origins of that sinister phrase some other time) in the process.

When she first started talking about "keto", I didn't really know what she meant, nor did I even care to. I just needed to know the rules and what I could and couldn't eat.

Her initial description of the plan sounded absurd to me, but I was fully interested in trying it out. After all, she had me at "you can eat all the bacon you want"! :D

The basic guidelines she gave me that day back in March (it's a rainy mid-December, in 2015, day as I write) were that I could eat all the fat and protein I wanted, but that I had to strictly limit carbs and sugars.

The goal was for me to eat no sugar grams and to keep my carb grams at under 30 for each day. 30 for the day! I had NO idea what that meant, until we got started with the plan.

I now realize that, prior to beginning this journey, it wasn't uncommon for me to eat 200 grams of carbs in a single meal! I had NO idea what a drastic change this was going to actually lead me to, but I went full into the plan.

Side Note, from 2017 now, dang it! (Procrastination SUX!) - I recently saw a post on Facebook that showed a popular Starbucks drink that had 87g of Carbs in it, and that's NOT very uncommon, unfortunately...

Prior to this year, my 45th on the planet, I had only attempted an actual "diet" once in my entire life! That experiment occurred in January of 2014, after reading a life changing book by the brilliant Tim Ferriss, called "The 4 Hour Work Week".

In this incredible book, Ferriss teaches us about the various experiments he has performed on himself and the results that followed. From there, he shares a diet that he calls the "slow carb" diet, which calls for one to eliminate all sugars, flours, and any other enriched, carby, starchy foods for 6 days a week. The diet allows for a "go hog wild" cheat day every 7th day!

This concept was right up my alley, as I loved the idea of having a free binge day that wouldn't impact my fitness objectives. I had, by that time, started feeling like my body was changing.

I was experiencing that bloated feeling much more often than I could recall in the past, and I was constantly gassy. It was actually so bad, that I was often quite embarrassed with the perpetual flatulent bombs that my dietary lifestyle were producing. It was bad and I was ready for a change!

Here I am again, the Time Traveler! It is April 22, 2017 as I Type this now, thoughts that come to mind: MAN, I used to fart a LOT!!! I really just don't anymore, unless I have a "Cheat Meal". Ketosis should be every woman's favorite Lifestyle, if for that reason alone! Loi ;)

The very first thing I did was to eliminate as much sugar from my diet as possible. I already mentioned my propensity to become the Cookie Monster, but I also had a much more consistent source of poisoning myself with sugar in the fact that I commonly drank 4-6 glasses of sweet tea per day!

I realized this only after the fact that I decided to drink only water for a few weeks in order to jumpstart this "slow carb" plan. The initial results were attention grabbing! I lost 17 lbs. in just 3 weeks!

I didn't know it then, but dropping out all that sugar was the true key to that rapid weight loss. I made a drastic change in my sugar intake, which was extremely high at that time, and my body responded immediately.

I was feeling pretty good about the weight loss and the inches coming off my waist, but I was still struggling with the bloating and gas. The slow carb diet calls for eating many beans and legumes, and that didn't do anything positive for my personal issues.

Over the course of a few months, I found myself drifting back to my old lifestyle of burgers, beer, pizza, and Mexican foods, and the "slow carb" plan just faded right out of my life.

I did pick up a great new positive habit during that process though, and it continues to pay dividends to this day. I never went back to sweet tea!

I started training myself to like unsweetened tea and now I actually love the flavor of it, so much so that I believe I now enjoy tea more than I ever have in my life. The stronger the better for me now! This alone has prevented me from many pounds of sugar consumption.

Did you know?

Americans consume an average of 66 POUNDS of sugar per year! It's no wonder that Diabetes and Obesity are so common these days.

It has truly become an epidemic of addiction in our fast food oriented society. We have become so addicted to sugars and carbs that most Americans can't even imagine a Low Carb lifestyle. I know I sure couldn't prior to March 2015!

There are numerous studies that indicate that concentrated sugars, the kind that are added into roughly 75% of packaged foods in the United States, create a chemical addiction in our brains. The addictive qualities of sugar, and its effects on brain chemistry, are comparable to that of heroin and cocaine!

My experience with Ketosis has been nothing short of rejuvenating, but I'd have never thought it possible prior to experiencing it. You see, the Keto (more accurately Low Carb/High Fat) Diet plan calls for a complete reversal of everything we've been taught to believe regarding nutrition.

I have been awakened to the Truth about how our government has cowed down to the food industry lobbyists, turning our nation's mindset on what is a "healthy diet" completely upside down! The famous "food pyramid", put out by the FDA and Government Health agencies, has us all brainwashed into demonizing fat, while edifying grains and wheat, which is completely backwards in regards to true health!

Because of the awakening that I have experienced, resulting from the phenomenal success of this dietary strategy, I am here to shine light on the Truth of what I've learned. It is my sincere hope that, through education and implementation, we can turn the tides on obesity, diabetes, and the myriad other health problems we have created with our poor dietary guidelines.

I pray that this book will help to illuminate for you that there are better ways to eat, which will free your body and mind to be the best you can be.

So let's see if I can do any justice to helping you understand the Keto Lifestyle and why you should consider giving it a go…

"Researchers have reported that the brain and central nervous system actually run more efficiently on ketones than they do on glucose." – Gary Taubes

Chapter 1

What is Ketosis?

Ketosis, as I have come to understand and love it, is a state in which the body burns FAT for FUEL! That concept alone just blows my mind! I was super intrigued, and very skeptical, the first time I heard this claim. The actual definition, according to Wikipedia:

"Ketosis /ki tousis/ is a metabolic state where most of the body's energy supply comes from ketone bodies in the blood, in contrast to a state of glycolysis, where blood glucose provides most of the energy."

To the unaware, a quick i-net search of "ketosis" will get you some scary sounding stuff! This is the first thing to pop up on MY search, back in 2015:

"a condition characterized by raised levels of ketone bodies in the body, associated with abnormal fat metabolism and diabetes mellitus."

"Abnormal fat metabolism and diabetes mellitus"!?? Who wants THAT!? Lol

Thankfully, there are people who have gone beyond these misleading definitions and discovered the amazing benefits that ketosis brings for the human body.

For the sake of those of you who want to know the science, I will briefly elaborate on exactly what IS ketosis, and I will provide additional resources later, for a more in depth study.

For the rest of you, you can skip this chapter if you want, knowing with full confidence that MY aforementioned definition will suffice for all your practical needs. Ketosis is a state in which the body burns fat for fuel. It's truly THAT simple!

Our bodies use three nutrients to create metabolic energy. Of the three nutrients (protein, carbohydrates, and fat) only carbohydrate is unnecessary. That's right, you read it correctly, your body has no NEED to ingest carbs!

When I first discovered this, I was extremely skeptical. However, with my wife's promises that I could eat all the bacon, brisket, and butter I wanted, I was totally willing to give it a try.

It turns out to be correct! When given the proper ratio of fat, carbs, and protein, the body will burn the fat for fuel, rather than storing it up for future use. The latter is how our body uses fat when we consume it in conjunction with carbs.

Another interesting quote from the Wiki article: "Longer-term ketosis may result from fasting or staying on a low-carbohydrate diet, and deliberately induced ketosis serves as a medical intervention for intractable epilepsy. In glycolysis, higher levels of insulin promote storage of body fat and block release of fat from adipose tissues, while in ketosis, fat reserves are readily released and consumed. For this reason, ketosis is sometimes referred to as the body's "fat burning" mode."

Scientifically, to the best of my understanding, the body is (due to our cultural diets) accustomed to "running" on glucose for energy, which it produces from carbohydrates.

Once broken down, the body uses what glucose it needs and then stores the rest in the liver. Fat, meanwhile, is stored for "emergency use" in various places in the body, including in and around organs.

"...the problem is that, in our overly fed society, "emergency use" never happens!" – Dr. Lee GreenTree

Each body-type varies, so there are different places that fat may be stored, but generally we know that men store predominantly in and around the abdomen (belly), while women tend to store along the hips and thighs (butt).

This storage of excess fat is what is causing the majority of health related problems in the US. We consume not only "too many" carbs, but we consume TOXIC levels of carbs in the form of sugars! But I digress, we will cover that in later chapters….

For our topic here, we need to know that the ketogenic body does *not* use glucose for energy, as it has been "deprived" (rather, re-trained!) from carbohydrates to the degree that it no longer needs them. The body *naturally* creates ketones in the blood and uses them for *direct* energy!

Fascinatingly enough, ketones actually provide MORE energy per measure than glucose!

While the Scientific Community, particularly the Medical Community, is still hesitant to proclaim this loudly, I have read *NUMEROUS* cases of studies that show all manner of bodily benefits from inducing a state of ketosis. We will discuss some of that in the next chapter.

There are some great places to get a more in depth look at the science behind ketosis, but I didn't want to regurgitate the fine work that those authors have already put forth.

I have given you *MY* summaries, based upon my first-hand *EXPERIENCE*, in conjunction with what I have learned through my own research and reading. I will point you to some of my favorite resources at the end of this book, for those of you who want to dig deeper.

"The belly rules the mind." – Spanish Proverb

Chapter 2

Why should one try to achieve Ketosis?

"A study with 23 Elderly with mild cognitive impairment showed that a ketogenic diet improved verbal memory performance after 6 weeks compared to a standard high carbohydrate diet. In a double-blind, placebo-controlled study, 152 patients with mild- to moderate Alzheimer's disease were given either a ketogenic agent or a placebo, while maintaining a normal diet. 90 days later, those receiving the drug showed marked cognitive improvement compared to placebo, which was correlated with the level of ketones in the blood." – from SA article:
http://blogs.scientificamerican.com/mind-guest-blog/the-fat-fueled-brain-unnatural-or-advantageous/

This is just one of MANY benefits that have been discovered about the effects of a ketogenic diet. I could probably fill a whole book just copying and pasting from all the research I have done, but I am really trying here to give you my personal perspective on why ketosis is worthy of a try.

I can't stress enough how it has changed my life for the better, but I will try to relay that to you in a manner that hopefully gets you moving towards your own better future and greater health.

As I mentioned in the introduction chapter, I was miserable with my diet prior to discovering Ketosis. I routinely over ate, and my carbohydrate intake was HUGE!

Prior to studying Ketosis, I never once even thought about how many carbs I ate, or ANY of my "macro" intake for that matter. In fact, prior to Keto (let's use pre-keto from here forward), I never even knew what "macros" were! I just simply had NO interest in being "healthy" by dietary modifications.

For those of you who may be like I was, "macros" are the term used to describe the big three that we talked about earlier: Protein, Carbohydrate, and Fat.

I now know just how important controlling my macros is to my overall health and well-being. I have truly enjoyed my keto-life, and it has *EVERYTHING* to do with knowing and adjusting the macro count.

As much as I still love the old Walton and Johnson skit, where they summarize the best way to lose weight, "eat less and move around more", it's much more scientific than that for much of our population.

For me, the biggest difference of all, aside from all the fat loss I've achieved, is the absence of the horrible cycle of over eating, only to be hungry again a few hours later.

I can now literally go all day without a single meal and feel totally fine, not "starving". I can also eat three to five keto meals and feel fine. In fact, the few times I have "over eaten" a keto meal have not left me feeling the misery that often accompanied a carb loaded meal.

I consider myself to have over eaten anytime I feel any kinda bulge or discomfort of "fullness" in my belly after a meal.

It just doesn't affect the body the same way. The science of that is that the blood sugar levels are very steady when in ketosis, whereas glucose (or sugar) burners are in a constant state of fluctuating blood sugar levels. This causes the "hunger pains"/cravings, so often experienced when eating carbohydrate heavy foods.

You too can benefit from a keto-lifestyle!

I encourage you to give it a try. What do you have to lose, besides fat!? Besides, you're not "losing" anything really. You are BURNING fat for FUEL!

Don't lose fat, USE fat! It's much more gratifying and satisfying, giving you unexpected, long lasting energy and focus, so that you can get more enjoyment out of life, while being in the best shape ever!

Give it a try! I think you'll be wonderfully surprised by how you look and feel after a few months of keto-living.

"Ketones are an efficient and effective fuel for human physiology without increasing the production of damaging free radicals. Ketosis allows a person to experience nonfluctuating energy throughout the day as well as enhanced brain function and possibly resistance to malignancy." – Dr. David Perlmutter

Chapter 3

How Does One Begin Producing Ketones?

The good news is that you don't have to DO anything to produce ketones, your body will naturally do that for you.

The bad news is that it WON'T do that until you sufficiently starve it of carbohydrate!

In order to generate ketones to the point of being "in ketosis" (commonly accepted as having blood ketone levels above .5 milomar), you will have to eliminate the stores of glucose in your liver, so that your body will be prompted to begin ketone production.

This can be accomplished by drastically lowering your carbohydrate consumption for an extended period of time. That time period will vary from person to person and by variances in your total carb counts.

For me, I targeted keeping my total carbohydrate count below 30 grams a day for one month. I found myself DRASTICALLY shedding weight, which I later learned was water weight; (we'll discuss that in future chapters) while simultaneously gaining unprecedented clarity and energy within just the first few weeks.

After becoming "keto adapted", which is the term commonly used to describe a person who is efficiently burning fat for fuel, I started noticing that I was hardly ever hungry.

I ate lots of my favorite foods, including brisket, barbacoa, avocado, butter, and cheeses, and the fat just melted from my body! The bloated feelings after eating were long gone, and neither I nor my family miss my former state of frequent flatulent that plagued the air around me!

Other notable improvements included higher energy levels, better sleep, improved libido and stamina, and a sense of clear mindedness unlike any other period in my life.

I can honestly say that, even without the dramatic fat loss, I would have gladly given up the carbs just for that short but profound list of results. Having noticed and felt these changes, I am quite convinced that my overall inner health has drastically improved during this process as well.

I have spoken to many friends, co-workers, and acquaintances, who all ask varying forms of the same questions. So here is my summation for how I would recommend embarking on training yourself to Use Fat for Fuel!

The first thing I would do is make sure you have some way of tracking what you consume. I highly recommend MyFitnessPal, which is an app that can be downloaded on any smartphone or tablet device.

I have no affiliations with this product or its creators, other than the fact that I used it constantly for the first six months or more of my own journey into ketosis.

By tracking exactly what you eat, you will do several things. Firstly, you will be more aware of your food choices, which helps to keep yourself "honest" and on track for your goals.

Secondly, you will be able to learn about the macros in each meal that you consume. This will help you, not only in counting your carbs, but so that you can learn patterns and the numbers associated with the various recipes you are eating, so that you can use what is working and change what doesn't. I will give you some exact examples in a later chapter…

As previously mentioned, I targeted a carb count of under 30 total grams per day when I first started my keto journey. Everything I have read up to this point supports that that is a good number to strive for.

Again, this may very well vary for some people, but I think it will be an effective number for the vast majority of people. I would suggest erring on the low side, rather than the high, if you truly want to get the most out of what Ketosis can do for you.

It is imperative that you eat enough Fat though. I have noticed that this is the hardest part of the diet. You actually have to seek out additional fat sources with each meal.

You should strive for 70-80% of your total caloric intake to be from Fat. Protein should be kept to around 15%, while Carbs should be no more than 5%.

Keeping these ratios intact, I have found, is more important than the actual counting of calories. The quantity of food intake will be regulated by your body, as you will cease to have the hunger pains and energy drops associated with a glucose based diet.

Once you have achieved Ketosis, and have learned how to measure your ketones, and are becoming in tune with your own body, then you can up the carb intake if you like.

I presently allow myself up to 60 grams per day, but still generally end up below 50. I have been adapted long enough now to be able to feel what is working and what drags me down.

You will get to that state as well, if you give it enough time and disciplined dedication. I am very excited for what you are going to experience!

Time Travel: from here in 2017, I now know that I haven't tracked or counted any macros in over a year. I have learned to be in tune with my body and my Ketosis comes naturally now. I just know what to eat and what not to, based upon the experience of having done so for over 2 years now. You too can get to that point. It is a truly liberating feeling!

In the next chapter, I am going to give you some exact snapshots of what meals I have eaten. You can then see my own patterns and put together your own.

Borrowing from the aforementioned Tim Ferris, I have found it extremely useful to create myself some staple, "go to" meals, so that I can stay disciplined and focused on my goals. I think that philosophy will work for anyone, you just have to convince yourself to give it a shot for a finite period of time.

I recall a quote from someone, but I don't recall whom, that said "I can put up with just about anything for a year"… lol, I'm sure I butchered that, and certainly don't know who to attribute it to, but I have adopted that mantra to get me through tough periods of "carb craving" at times.

The good news is that it doesn't take a year. You can most likely achieve ketosis within the first 3 - 6 weeks, if you are diligent in your disciplining yourself on what you consume.

You can set up the period goal, I would suggest taking it weekly at first, but having a first milestone set for one month.

If you can keep your carbs down for one month, while keeping balance with your protein and fat intake (which we'll get more specific about in later chapters), then I believe you will be flat out amazed at what your body will do for you in Ketosis. Let's get started!

"Nothing would be more tiresome than eating and drinking if God had not made them a pleasure as well as a necessity." – Voltaire

Chapter 4

Action Plan

Alright, time for breakfast! Mmmm, I smell BACON!!! :D

Yup, there's just something about the smell of bacon in the morning! It's one of the few things that actually make me happy to jump out of bed. I am NO kinda "morning person", but when my wife has the house smelling like bacon, well, sleepy time is over!

A wonderful keto-breakfast can be had with 3 or 4 eggs, cooked in bacon grease, butter, and/or olive oil. *I sometime use all three fats in the pan, creating wonderfully delicious eggs…* Add some garlic and onions to the oils, then cook your eggs right in with it, however you like them!

I like mine soft scrambled, mixed into the pan, rather than beaten. Bury them in an avalanche of your favorite cheeses and cover the pan for a few minutes to let it melt. Then, add some sliced avocado and several slices of bacon, cooked to your liking, and you'll be good to go!

When I first started this diet, I could physically eat much more than I can today. There's something to the difference in how one feels when satiated with healthy fats, verses being burdened with sugars and carbs that weigh down the body's inner workings and cause an overall sluggish, lethargic feeling.

I have noticed drastic changes in my own eating habits, in that I eat substantially smaller portions now (not at first, it took some time to adjust) yet I feel much more satisfied and that feeling lasts hours longer than when I was eating carbs and sugars!

As I mentioned before, this has mainly to do with the sugar levels in the blood. The stabilized glucose levels prevent spikes and thus limit cravings and hunger pains, leaving me much more satisfied.

Back to food now!

You may find yourself needing an adjustment period during your transition. Having gone through this stage without really knowing what to expect, I can say that it would have been easier on me if I had been better prepared.

I think it's a wise strategy to find 3 or 4 main meal platforms that can be either directly duplicated or just tweaked here and there for variety satisfaction. I would do something like this:

Breakfast: we mentioned a pretty good one above. You can take that base of meat and fat and add some spinach if you like, for fiber and bulk. You can substitute your own favorite meat, or have (blaspheme for those of us born in Texas) no meat at all.

Just be sure you are eating enough fat. Avocados are a wonderful source for that! In addition to the butter, olive oil, and bacon grease I mentioned earlier, I use a lot of coconut oil as well.

Coconut is one of Nature's absolute best sources of fat. In fact, it may be THE best source of fat for us, but there is still much ongoing scientific research on that. Suffice it to say that it is a wonderful source of fat for the keto dieter.

It's so useful, that I have actually been working to develop a line of keto-friendly products from coconut sources. If those things come to fruition in time, I will provide you with links so that you can benefit from these products in your own diet.

As of now, we are just Developing, but the reason for the inspiration comes from the fact that I have been creating shakes out of a low carb protein powder, combined with almond or cashew milk, and mixed with heavy whipping cream. This makes for a fast, efficient, on the go meal replacement, but is a bit tedious to mix it all up in the proper ratios and such.

I hope to simplify that with a keto-shake type product that will contain the proper balances we need for our keto lifestyles... stay tuned for more there!

Now, Let's Do Lunch!

I live in Texas, and in Texas, we love our BBQ! I happen to be a veteran of the pro BBQ circuit, from my younger days, so I myself am very fond of BBQ. In fact, as I mentioned before, it's probably my affinity for brisket that got me started down this path of Ketosis to begin with!

You see, it's just flat out hard to beat a nice, fatty cut of moist, slow smoked brisket! It's like a little slice of Heaven here on Earth, but it packs a punch full of fat and calories.

It's very easy to get overweight when eating traditional BBQ fare, which would include bread, potato salad, beans, etc… all of which combine to create a huge caloric count that overloads the body's ability to make proper use of it all.

It's no wonder we have such a plague of obesity and a general population that is in such poor health. But don't worry! Ketosis provides for us a solution that turns what would be a terrible meal in the aforementioned BBQ menu, to a powerhouse of flavor and optimal fuel for your body!

"Use Fat" never sounded as good as when one gets that first bite of fatty brisket! Mmmm, mmm, GOOD!

I definitely went off on a tangent there, but for lunch, you guessed it… brisket! I often order a half pound of fatty or "moist cut" brisket for my lunch. I skip the sides, unless I'm in the mood for some greens or a salad or something.

Sometimes I'll get some sausage or pulled pork, but mostly I'm good with that tender, moist, marbled brisket, that just melts in your mouth!

I have even, on occasion, been known to slather a few pats of butter onto the sliced brisket, which really gives it a nice fat boost and provides my body with optimal energy levels!

I really do LOVE this "diet"!!! :D

Perhaps the only thing more common in Texas than BBQ is Mexican food. We have even claimed our own sub variety of it, known as Tex-Mex. Now I truly LOVE Mexican food, but most plates, whether authentic or Tex-Mex, are heavily loaded with carbs!

From the moment you sit down, at just about any Mexican restaurant you will find, you are given heaping baskets full of yummy, greasy corn chips, which can pack a whopping 2g of carbs PER CHIP!

Yes, you read that correctly. EACH chip contains approximately 2 grams of carbs and, since they are a corn based product, will also add significantly to your total sugar intake!

As I mentioned earlier, it was far from uncommon for me to frequent Mexican restaurants and, when I did, I would consume an average of 2 – 3 BASKETS full of those salty little devils!

It's no wonder I was so heavy laden with fat in my body composition! Which, by the way, as I write on August 1, 2016, is down to 16%, from the 27% that I started out in back in January of 2015!

Time Traveler Update – I'm a lean (13% body fat) 155lbs now, down from pushing at 200lbs before Ketosis!

Needless to say, I avoid those chips now. If I'm by myself, I just ask the wait person to not even bother bringing them out, thus eliminating the temptation for me.

If I'm with someone else, who is eating the chips, I will occasionally have one or two, but I am really good at not going beyond 3, as it's just not worth the carb count to me.

Mexican food is still very much a staple of my diet, I just had to make some adjustments. Aside from the aforementioned chips, I avoid the rice and beans, and I rarely eat tortillas, though I do sometimes allow myself the 16g of carb for a breakfast taco treat!

On those days, I just buckle down and really watch my carb consumption for the remainder of the day. Sometimes I won't even eat again (and am not really even hungry) on a day in which I've allowed myself a couple of breakfast tacos.

Most times I just order the meats that I love, barbacoa, pastor, chicharron, etc, as a-la-carte dishes in and of themselves. I commonly will order 2 barbacoa and 2 pastor "tacos" with no tortillas.

I often add the Mexican salad, consisting of lettuce, pico-de-gallo, and some lime for flavoring. I add cheese and sliced avocado, to increase the fat grams, and it is wonderfully satisfying. I eat this meal combination several times weekly and it is my most common food source.

Experiment with the different meats that you yourself like and don't be afraid to try new things, like the chicharron, but beware that is often a very spicy dish!

Remember to always add the avocado, as this is a prime source of fat for your body. You can also add Mexican sour cream where available, which will give a little extra fat and a lot of extra flavor. Enjoy!

Dinner time usually finds me not very hungry, so I often just have another shake, or something light, like say a salad with lots of blue cheese crumbles and blue cheese dressing!

NOTE HERE: Be careful and read labels closely! The food companies like to hide sugars everywhere they can! Pay attention to the carb counts of course, but also watch out for the sugars hidden in the ingredients list, because they don't always show up in the sugar measurements on the nutritional panel. They have gotten very sneaky regarding that type of thing!

According to sugarsicence.org, a website dedicated to helping consumers control their sugar consumption and educate themselves on the harmful facts regarding too much sugar in the diet, there are over 61 alternate names for sugar hiding in our food labels. Sixty One!!

Some hidden sugars they list to watch out for include agave nectar, barley malt, buttered syrup, cane juice, cane juice crystals, caramel, carob syrup, corn sweetener, corn syrup, dextrin, dextrose, fruit juice, glucose, golden syrup, honey, malt syrup, maltodextrin, maltol, maltose, mannose, molasses, muscovado, panocha, refiner's syrup, rice syrup, saccharose, sorghum syrup, sucrose sweet sorghum, syrup, treacle, etc… There are many, many more, but I left off the obvious ones that contained the word "sugar" in the product name.

You can read more about alternate names for sugar at the aforementioned website of **www.sugarscience.org/hidden-in-plain-sight/**

In short, when deciding which salad dressing to use, try to find yourself a brand that has few ingredients and NO sugars, whenever possible.

"A long habit of not thinking a thing wrong, gives it a superficial appearance of being right, and raises at first a formidable outcry in defense of custom. But the tumult soon subsides. Time makes more converts than reason." - Thomas Paine, *Common Sense*

Chapter 5

Some History, Some Math, Some Common Sense

Alright, now I am quite sure that there will be some of you who, like me, want to learn everything you can about things that interest you.

I hope, if I've accomplished my goal of peeking your interest in a low carb/high fat lifestyle, that you are now at least interested in knowing more about ketosis. Here are some more insights into some of the History and Science behind this Concept.

Human beings were created (yes, I said "created", but that's an entirely different book than this one) with a very unique biology.

We are, in fact, the most unique creatures on Earth, in that we alone have tremendous powers of creativity, cognition, drive, and self-awareness, which enable us to impact all of Life, through our constant scientific breakthroughs and technological advances.

Throughout the thousands of years of Human History, our genetic makeup has been the same as when we were first created, but our food sources change almost daily these days, and have been doing so for several decades now. Consequently, there is nothing "new" about this dietary recommendation that I am advocating to you.

What's "new" is that, for perhaps the first era in our History, we now have so much available Data to us that even laymen, such as myself, can become highly educated on just about any given topic of interest, by digging through the World Wide Web (of sometimes confusing, often tainted and manipulated by "the Powers That Be", information and stories...) to sift the accumulated Knowledge, so that it can be compared with one's actual experience(s).

I have been doing that for years on topics that I enjoy learning about, of which there are many that I would trade all that time and energy back for the opportunity to pursue other things. Not this one though!

I truly feel blessed (and now obligated to Share) to have found something so Life-Changing, Confirmable, Practical, Universal, and Logical, that just about anyone can DO to improve their overall Quality of Life.

I thank God daily for allowing me to feel so refreshed, satisfied, energetic, and happy with my choice of Diet. That being said, I did dig around a bit when I first started learning about how to "do" Ketosis.

In my studies, the oldest mention I could find of this type of Food Philosophy came out of England in the late 1800's. 1863 to be exact!

In May of 1863, William Banting, an English undertaker by Trade, published a pamphlet on what he believed to be the "correct way" to eat. He was 67 years old at the time, and had been through many failed diets and trends, having battled with obesity for most of his life.

Once he figured out the formula, and had success in applying it, he wrote his "Letter on Corpulence, Addressed to the Public", which can still be found and read for free!

Here is a link for your enjoyment:
https://archive.org/details/letteroncorpulen00bant

I am particularly fond of the way Englishmen wrote back in that time and era… Should you not wish to read the entire thing, although it is rather short and fun to read, I will sum up for you, in three words, the most important thing he did to free himself from "Corpulence". **Eat less sugar!**

He describes for us how he went from 202lbs. to 167lbs., and credits that "diminution of something like 1 lb. per week" to having cut back on bread, milk, butter, beer, sugar, and potatoes…"

I remind you, this was in 1863, so combining that information with what we now know about the effects of those things on the body, it becomes evident that the bread, sugar, beer, and potatoes were indeed terrible for him. However, he could have kept all the butter and most of the milk. As we have already discussed above.

The point of this particular Storyline is that "Banting", as it became known in later years, is the oldest mention that I could find for reducing these certain things from one's diet.

It should be noted that there was not the proliferation of mass produced food sources that we enjoy as both a Blessing and a Curse in our world today, and we certainly weren't being bombarded by images and ads for all the sugary garbage that has become so much of the Staple food sources for our Society.

Did you know? *A normal can of Soda contains more sugar than most people would have consumed in an entire year, just a few hundred years ago!??*

An interesting math problem!

Remember the Macros that I told you about earlier? As promised, I want to touch on some important things about Energy.

Of the three Macros, Protein, Carbohydrate (Carbs), and Fat, only Fat differs on the caloric count per gram. Each gram of Fat produces 9 Calories, while each gram of Carbs and Protein produce only 4.

When one looks at that from a "calorie counting" standpoint, which you will have noticed had NOTHING to do with anything that I have been doing or talking about, it would seem that Fat would be the "bad guy", as it has very well been relegated to. This, however, would be the WRONG way to look at this little miracle of Creation!

The RIGHT way to view this is that for every gram ingested, Fat gives you more than twice the Energy/Fuel that your body burns than do Carbs or Proteins! That's a really radical thing to ponder, especially when combined with another fact that I discovered...

Ever heard of the old expression, "Carb-up"? Marathoners and other Endurance Athletes (remember, my wife is very much into that stuff) often use this tactic to prepare themselves for their races or events. It is actually impossible for us to store more than 2000 calories worth of Carbohydrate, within our body, at any given time. This means that Endurance Athletes have to continue to feed themselves Carbs, during their event(s), in order to prevent a performance drop.

Even while eating, the body can only digest and process about 60 grams per hour, so that would be the equivalent of about 240 calories. That's 240 Units of Energy that they would have available to them, per hour, to complete the event.

A body that burns fat for fuel has tens of thousands of calories ready at a moment's notice!

Remember that "Emergency Use" we mentioned earlier? Well, here's where it comes into play very nicely. Our bodies naturally store Fat, even if we don't show it on the outside. It is readily available from many organs and cells within us, to the degree that even a well-trained, lean athlete, can hold 10,000 calories of Fat within his body at any given time!

In order for that to be readily available to burn, without the body first trying to compensate for its energy deficiency by lowering performance, the athlete would have to have become keto-adapted. Therefore, it stands to reason that being in Ketosis is ideal for someone who has large expenditures of energy, and needs a steady, readily available supply of fuel for his body.

Keto provides that fuel! Burn Fat for Fuel! ☺ Has a nice ring to it, don't you think?

If you are still with me, I hope that I have provided for you a genuine desire to learn more about how your body uses food, and specifically how Fat can be your best friend, rather than the demon it has been made out to be by our commercialized culture.

I suspect that, very soon, the wave of Truth regarding Ketosis and the benefits of a Low Carb/High Fat diet/lifestyle will begin to turn the tide against the lies and misconceptions that we have been taught to believe.

I think it is very important that we continue to educate ourselves on all aspects of Life, not just Diet, rather than to just accept things and float along, consuming all that's placed before us without a moment's hesitation or thought.

"I have seen mood stabilization, reduced or eliminated depression, reduced or eliminated anxiety, improved cognitive functioning, greatly enhanced and evened-out energy levels, cessation of seizures, improved overall neurological stability, cessation of migraines, improved sleep, improvement in autistic symptoms, improvements with PCOS (polycystic ovary syndrome), improved gastrointestinal functioning, healthy weight loss, cancer remissions and tumor shrinkage, much better management of underlying previous health issues, improved symptoms and quality of life in those struggling with various forms of autoimmunity (including many with type 1 and 1.5 diabetes), fewer colds and flus, total reversal of chronic fatigue, improved memory, sharpened cognitive functioning, and significantly stabilized temperament. And there is quality evidence to support the beneficial impact of a fat-based ketogenic approach in all these types of issues" – Nora Gedgaudas, as quoted in *"Keto Clarity: Your Definitive Guide to the Benefits of a Low-Carb,*

High-Fat Diet" by Jimmy Moore and Eric Westman

Summation and Useful Resources

I hope I have gotten your attention well enough to at least cause you to give it a try. I challenge you, and you will thank me for it if you try it, to check it out for yourself. Please remember though, I'm just a guy who Burns Fat for Fuel. I am NOT a doctor, nor even a Nutritionist or Trainer.

I am actually quite averse to exercise for the sake of exercise, and prefer to stay active by doing things that I love to do, such as hiking, fishing, exploring, and playing with my many children.

So, with that said, please do consult your doctor if you have ever had any problems with your Pancreas or are Diabetic.

Diabetes is one of the things that can be drastically improved by adopting a Keto Lifestyle, but you must be careful to ensure that you are getting the proper amounts of Fat in your diet.

It is easy to get too much Protein, and not enough Fat consumption when first starting out, which is why I recommend a tracking system of some kind. As I mentioned before, I used "MyFitnessPal" app when I first started out. There are probably dozens of such resources available now, so find one that works best for you.

Here are some of the resources that I have enjoyed. I hope they bless you.

Recommended Books:

"Cholesterol Clarity: What the HDL Is Wrong With My Numbers?" by Jimmy Moore, and Dr. Eric Westman

"Keto Clarity: Your Definitive Guide to the Benefits of a Low-Carb, High-Fat Diet" by Jimmy Moore, and Dr. Eric Westman

"Grain Brain: The Surprising Truth about Wheat, Carbs, and Sugar – Your Brain's Silent Killers" by Dr. David Perlmutter
IF you only read one book on dietary health for the rest of your life, PLEASE let it be this one! Dr. Perlmutter provides eye opening information here that should be, IMO, "Required Reading" for anyone in the Healthcare/Nutritional Fields.

"The Art and Science of Low Carbohydrate Performance" by Stephen Phinney and Jeff Volek

"Good Calories, Bad Calories: Challenging the Conventional Wisdom on Diet, Weight Control, and Disease" – by Gary Taubes

Movies:

Fed Up – by Stephanie Soechtig
Super Size Me – by Morgan Spurlock

Websites:
www.ruled.me.com
www.sugarscience.org
www.burnfatforfuel.com

Afterword

I first started writing this book back in November of 2015, but I actually had less than 1,000 words written by August of 2016.

Back then, I was very excited to "tell the world" about this "new diet" that I had found, but "Writing" was something new to me. So, though I immersed myself in education and research, there was very little information, even on the web, to be found on Ketosis back then.

Now (April of 2017) "keto" is a common buzz word thrown about all over the web and social media sites. It has become quite the "new thing", as I suspected it would after I experienced my own amazing results.

I have experienced a dramatic transformation from body fat loss. Friends, family, and associates are constantly asking me, "what did you do?" and "how can I do it?", so I wanted to complete this book, so as to give an overview of Keto Theory and to point you on the direction of increasing your knowledge of the subject. I hope it finds you well.

I, as is my usual tendency, did much procrastinating over getting anything typed out, but I did a ton of reading and lots of experimenting with the diet and all aspects of its influences.

I can still say, with confidence, that it is hands down the best, most healthy way of eating that I have ever tried in my 45 plus years of living. With that said, please do take precautions and seek a doctor's advice if you plan on putting any minor children on this diet.

Our 14 year old son, who has Duchenne Muscular Dystrophy, spent a week in the Pediatric ICU because his pancreas couldn't handle the sudden change in dietary fat!

It was a grueling, stressful, and scary situation that I wouldn't wish on anyone. I recommend going slowly and checking with your doctor if you have any questions or concerns about living a Low Carb/High Fat diet.

I wish you all the best and I welcome your questions and feedback at
www.iBurnFatForFuel.com

Twitter: @FatBurnerKMB

Facebook: Red Oak Nutrition

God's blessings to you and your family.

With Love,
kmb – April 22, 2017 – Houston, TX

About The Author:

Kevin lives in Houston, TX with his wife and children. They have 7 children, 2 dogs, and a cat named Merlin. He enjoys music, reading, chess, and travel.

He is presently working on a few, soon to be published, novels, including "The Weaver", "Transparent Man", and "J.A.R. Heads"

You can follow him on Twitter at "@fatburnerkmb" Or find his blog at
www.TooManyOpenWindows.com

Kevin's number one goal in life is to spread the Love of Christ to all whom he can reach, in Story or in Action… Be Blessed.

><)))>

www.ingramcontent.com/pod-product-compliance
Lightning Source LLC
Chambersburg PA
CBHW071241280526
45788CB00004B/1531